DEDICATION

I dedicated this book to everyone who has the zeal to help or even help cancer patients, either with his money, advice; or even showing love to them. May God bless them all.

PREFACE

I wrote this book to help
people know a little bit about
cancer so that they know what
causes it, and what to avoid
especially in our daily meals,
you may find out that some
food is dangerous to our
health but we don't know. So,
in this book, we will know
what to eat and what to
eliminate. Also, to remind
those that have the disease
what God says about it,
whether you are a Christian
or Muslim; if you have this

kind of disease or any disease in particular; it doesn't mean that God didn't love you, He loves you and he has a great reward for you in the hereafter, if you endure and accept your destiny. Please be patient, by God's' grace God will guide you and help you out of every hardness and sorrow.

TABLE OF CONTENTS

1. MEANING OF CANCER
2. DIFFERENCE BETWEEN NORMAL CELL AND CANCER CELL
3. TYPES OF CANCER
4. HOW CANCER SPREAD
5. CAUSES OF CANCER
6. SIGNS OF CANCER
7. SOME FOOD THAT CAN CAUSE CANCER
8. PREVENTIVE FOODS FOR CANCER
9. CANCER TREATMENTS
10. HOW TO COPE WITH CANCER DIAGNOSIS

11. SOME RELAXATION TECHNIQUES THAT MAY BE HELPFUL

12. HOW TO PREVENT CANCER

13. WHAT QUR'AN SAYS ABOUT ENDURING DURING HARDSHIP

14. WHAT BIBLE SAYS ABOUT PATIENCE

15. CONCLUSION

CANCER

Cancer is a disease in which some of the body's cells grow uncontrollably and spread to other parts of the body. Cancer can start almost anywhere in the human body, which is made up of trillions of cells. Normally, human cells grow and multiply (through a process called cell division) to form new cells as the body needs them. When cells grow old or become damaged, they die, and new cells take their place. Sometimes this orderly process breaks down, and abnormal or damaged cells grow and multiply when they shouldn't. These cells may form tumors, which are lumps of tissue. Tumors can be

cancerous or not cancerous (benign). Cancerous tumors spread into, or invade, nearby tissues and can travel to distant places in the body to form new tumors (a process called metastasis). Cancerous tumors may also be called malignant tumors. Many cancers form solid tumors, but cancers of the blood, such as leukemias, generally do not. Benign tumors do not spread into, or invade, nearby tissues. When removed, benign tumors usually don't grow back, whereas cancerous tumors sometimes do. Benign tumors can sometimes be quite large, however. Some can cause serious symptoms or be life-threatening, such as benign tumors in the brain.

DIFFERENCES BETWEEN NORMAL CELLS AND CANCER CELLS

Cancer cells differ from normal cells in many ways. For instance, cancer cells:

. Grow in the absence of signals telling them to grow. Normal cells only grow when they receive such signals.

. Ignore signals that normally tell cells to stop dividing or to die (a process known as programmed cell death or apoptosis).

. Invade into nearby areas and spread to other areas of the body. Normal cells stop growing when they encounter other cells, and most normal cells do not move around the body.

. Tell blood vessels to grow toward tumors. These blood vessels supply tumors with oxygen and nutrients and remove waste products from tumors.

. Hide from the immune system. please the immune system normally eliminates damaged or abnormal cells.

. Trick the immune system into helping cancer cells stay alive and grow. For instance, some cancer cells convince immune cells to protect the tumor instead of attacking it.

. Accumulate multiple changes in their chromosomes, such as duplications and deletions of chromosome parts. Some cancer cells have double the normal number of chromosomes.

. Rely on different kinds of nutrients than normal cells. In addition, some cancer cells make energy from nutrients in a different way than most normal cells. This lets cancer cells grow more quickly.

TYPES OF CANCER

Doctors divide cancer into types based on where it begins. Four main types of cancer are:

. SARCOMAS

SARCOMAS; A sarcoma begins in the tissues that support and connect the body.

A sarcoma can develop in fat, muscles, nerves, tendons, joints, blood vessels, lymph vessels, cartilage, or bone

. CARCINOMAS

CARCINOMA; A
carcinoma begins in the skin or the tissue that covers the surface of internal organs and glands. Carcinomas usually form solid tumors. They are the most common type of cancer. Examples of carcinomas include prostate cancer, breast cancer, lung cancer, and colorectal cancer.

. LEUKEMIA

LEUKEMIA: Leukemia is a cancer of the blood. Leukemia begins when healthy blood cells change and grow uncontrollably. The 4 main types of leukemia are acute lymphocytic leukemia, chronic lymphocytic leukemia, acute myeloid leukemia, and chronic myeloid leukemia.

. LYMPHOMAS

LYMPHOMAS: Lymphoma is a cancer that begins in the lymphatic system. The lymphatic system is a network of vessels and glands that help fight infection. There are

2 main types of lymphomas:
Hodgkin lymphoma and non-
Hodgkin lymphoma. There
are many other types of
cancer.

HOW CANCER SPREADS

As a cancerous tumor grows,
the bloodstream or lymphatic
system may carry cancer cells
to other parts of the body.
During this process, the
cancer cells grow and may
develop into new tumors. This
is known as metastasis.

One of the first places cancer often spreads is to the lymph nodes. Lymph nodes are tiny, bean-shaped organs that help fight infection. They are located in clusters in different parts of the body, such as the neck, groin area, and under the arms.

Cancer may also spread through the bloodstream to distant parts of the body. These parts may include the bones, liver, lungs, or brain. Even if the cancer spreads, it is still named for the area where it began. For example, if breast cancer spreads to the lungs, it is called metastatic breast cancer, not lung cancer.

CAUSES OF CANCER

The main cause of cancer is mutations or changes to the DNA in your cells. Genetic mutations can be inherited. They can also occur after birth as a result of environmental forces.

These external causes, are called *CARCINOGENS* and can include:

CARCINOGENS; A carcinogen is any substance, radionuclide, or radiation that promotes carcinogenesis, which is the formation of cancer Carcinogens can be classified as genotoxic or nongenotoxic. Genotoxins cause irreversible genetic damage or mutations by braiding to DNA. The genotoxins (chemical agents) like N-nitroso-N-methyl urea (NMU) or non-chemical agents such as ultraviolet light and ionizing radiation. Carcinogens are not necessarily immediately toxic; thus, their effect can be insidious. **The carcinogens may increase the risk of**

cancer by altering cellular metabolism or damaging DNA directly in cells, which interferes with biological processes and induces uncontrolled malignant division, ultimately leading to the formation of tumors

. PHYSICAL CARCINOGENS RADIATION AND ULTRAVIOLET (UV) LIGHT; is the most prominent and ubiquitous physical carcinogen in our natural environment. It is highly genotoxic but does not penetrate the body any deeper than the skin. Like all organisms regularly exposed to sunlight, the human skin is extremely well adapted to continuous UV stress.

. CHEMICAL CARCINOGENS; like cigarette smoke, asbestos, alcohol, air pollution, and contaminated food and drinking water.

. BIOLOGICAL CARCINOGENS; are like viruses, bacteria, and parasites

According to the WHO (World Health Organization) Trusted Source, about 33 percent of cancer deaths may be caused by tobacco, alcohol, high body mass index (BMI), low fruit and vegetable consumption, and not getting enough physical activity.

SIGNS OF CANCER

The common signs and symptoms of cancer in both men and women don't mean that whenever you see any of these signs is a cancer please kindly go and see your doctor first. the signs are:

1)PAIN; Bone cancer often hurts from the beginning. Some brain tumors cause headaches that last for days and don't get better with treatment. Pain can also be a late sign of cancer, so see a doctor if you don't know why it's happening or if it doesn't go away.

2)WEIGHT LOSS WITHOUT TRYING; Almost half of people who have cancer lose weight. It's often one of the signs that they notice first.

3)FATIGUE; If you're tired all the time and rest doesn't help, tell your doctor.
Leukemia often wears you out, or you could have blood loss from colon or stomach cancer. Cancer-related weight

loss can leave you exhausted, too.

4)FEVER; If it's high or lasts more than 3 days, call your doctor. Some blood cancers, like lymphoma, cause a fever for days or even weeks.

5)CHANGES IN YOUR SKIN; Have your doctor look at unusual or new moles, bumps, or marks on your body to be sure skin cancer isn't lurking. Your skin can also provide clues to other kinds of cancers. If it's darkened, looks yellow or red, itches, or sprouts more hair, or if you have an unexplained rash, it could be a sign of

liver, ovarian, or kidney
cancer or lymphoma.

6)SORES THAT DON'T
HEAL; Spots that bleed and
won't go away are also signs
of skin cancer. Oral cancer
can start as sores in your
mouth. If you smoke, chew
tobacco, or drink a lot of
alcohol, you're at higher risk.

7)COUGH OR HOARSENESS
THAT DOESN'T GO AWAY; A
cough is one sign of lung
cancer, and hoarseness may
mean cancer of your voice box
(larynx) or thyroid gland.

8)UNUSUAL
BLEEDING; Cancer can make

blood show up where it shouldn't be. Blood in your poop is a symptom of colon or rectal cancer. And tumors along your urinary tract can cause blood in your urine.

9)ANEMIA; This is when your body doesn't have enough red blood cells, which are made in your bone marrow. Cancers like leukemia, lymphoma, and multiple myeloma can damage your marrow. Tumors that spread there from other places might

SOME FOODS THAT CAN CAUSE CANCER

Your health is your best asset, and your diet can have a huge impact on it. You probably have a general idea of which foods you should be eating vegetables, fruits, whole grains, and fish but what about which ones to avoid? Here's a list of 16 potentially cancer-causing foods.

1.CANNED TOMATOES; The cans of foods are typically lined with bisphenol-a (BPA), a chemical that has been linked to cancer and other serious health problems. Because they're so acidic, tomatoes are more likely to leech problematic levels of BPA from the can into the food. Stick to fresh tomatoes to avoid contamination.

2.REFINED SUGAR;
According to the research conducted way back in 1931 sugar provides fuel for tumors, allowing them to grow in size. In addition to wreaking havoc on your metabolism, processed sugars may be more readily accessible to cancer cells. Cancer Treatment Centers of America explores the effects

of different types of sugar on the body.

3.ALCOHOL; Although moderate consumption can lower your risk of heart disease, alcohol abuse is the leading cause of cancer behind tobacco use. A meta-analysis of drinking and cancer risk found an association between heavy drinking and an increased risk of mouth, colon, liver, and other cancers.

4.FRENCH FRIES AND POTATO CHIPS; Acrylamide, a chemical used in certain industrial processes that's also found in cigarette smoke, can form in starchy foods like potatoes when they're cooked at high temperatures. While more research is needed, the American Cancer Society supports continued evaluation of acrylamide and its effects.

5.PROCESSED MEAT; The International Agency for Research on Cancer (IARC) classified processed meat as a carcinogen after experts from 10 countries looking at more than 800 studies found eating 50 grams of four strips of bacon or one hot dog every day increased the risk of colorectal cancer by 18 percent.

6.MASS PRODUCED BREAD;
Potassium bromate, a food
additive used to make bread
dough more elastic, has been
identified as a possible
carcinogen by many health
organizations and is United
States, California requires a
warning label for products
containing this ingredient,
which is sometimes listed as
brominated flour.

7.ARTIFICIAL COLORS; A
2010 report by the Center for
Science in the Public Interest
called Food Dies: A rainbow of
risks concluded the nine FDA-
approved artificial dyes
approved in the United States
may be carcinogenic, cause

behavior problems, and/or are inadequately tested.

8.MICROWAVE POPCORN; Some microwave popcorn bags are lined with a chemical that decomposes to produce perfluorooctanoic acid (PFOA). PFOA has been linked to an increased risk of liver, prostate, and other cancers. Another chemical used in artificial butter flavor, diacetyl, may cause lung damage. It's easy to make your own microwave popcorn with a brown paper bag and some coconut oil.

9.HYDROGENATED OILS; In addition to being bad for your

heart, hydrogenated oils can cause inflammation and cell damage that has been linked to cancer and other diseases. The U.S. Food and Drug Administration banned partially hydrogenated oils in January of 2015, giving food manufacturers three years to remove them from their products.

10.CHARRED MEAT; The high temperatures used to heavily grill meat can produce carcinogens called heterocyclic aromatic amines and polycyclic aromatic hydrocarbons if you like your steak Well done.

11.FARMED SALMON;
Salmon raised on farms are
more likely to be
contaminated by carcinogens.
According to the
environmental working
group, farmed salmon have 16
times the polychlorinated
biphenyls (PCBs) found in
wild salmon.

12.SODA (Or "Pop" if you're
from the Midwest); A Swedish
study found men who drank
one 11-oz. soda a day were
40% more likely to develop
prostate cancer. An
analysis by Johns Hopkins
University in Maryland and
US Consumer Reports found
an association between 4-

methylimidazole, the chemical that gives some soda its caramel color, and increased cancer risk.

13.RED MEAT; The World Health Organization's International Agency for Research on Cancer has classified red meat as probably carcinogenic to humans based on evidence showing a link between its consumption and the development of colorectal cancer.

14.TOO MUCH PASTA; Pasta, bagels, and other "white" carbohydrates have a high glycemic index (GI), meaning they more rapidly elevate blood sugar levels. A recent study showed people whose diets had a high GI had a 49 percent greater risk of being diagnosed with lung cancer. Adding healthy fats (like olive oil) and protein to pasta helps lower the overall glycemic index of the meal it is a part of. Some pasta, like Braille Protein Plus, has a lower glycemic index.

15.MILK; 2004 meta-analysis found a positive association between milk consumption and prostate cancer. Some experts believe the animal fat in dairy products may increase cancer risk.

16.GENETICALLY-MODIFIED ORGANISMS (GMOs); Studies indicate an association between GMOs and the chemicals used to grow them and the development of tumors.

PREVENTIVE FOODS FOR CANCER

1.GARLIC: The active principle in garlic, allicin is the secret ingredient that fights against cancer, especially colorectal, prostate and stomach cancer. Allicin can also be found in other foods such as onions, chives, and leeks. Including 2-5 grams of fresh garlic in your meals by spicing up your sauce or dry roasting your meat with the pungent food ensures sufficient daily intake. Just be sure to take your burps away from the dining table.

2.OLIVE OIL: It's been quite a while since doctors and fitness specialists have been stressing using olive oil as the go-to medium for cooking. It sure has truckloads of health benefits. One of these benefits is decreasing the risk of cancer in various parts of the body like the digestive system, colorectal area, and breasts. Sprinkle some over your salads or cook your veggies and meat in it, olive oil is surely a great cancer fighter.

3.BERRIES: Berries are rich in antioxidants which help fight free radicals that can cause cancer. Black raspberries, in particular, wick contain a plant pigment called anthocyanin's which have antioxidative properties. They especially decrease the risk of colorectal cancer, oral cancer and esophageal cancer when consumed.

4.FLAXSEED: Flaxseeds provide a lot of crunch in the fight against cancer. Rich in fiber and unsaturated fats, flaxseeds also kill cancer cells and restricts cancer growth in the breast, colorectum, and prostate. Roast flaxseeds and pound them into a powder to sprinkle on your breakfast cereal or salad, munch on them as is, or top your smoothie with them to boost your body in smacking down the disease.

5.SOY: Soy is a plant-based 'superfood' which is rich in

proteins, unsaturated fats, vitamin, minerals and antioxidants. The antioxidant isoflavone present in tofu, soy milk, soy nuts and soya chunks help prevent low density lipoprotein (LDL) from giving you bad cholesterol, keeping diseases like obesity and heart-related illnesses at bay. It also helps reduce the risk of breast cancer tremendously.

6.BROCCOLI: broccoli contains isothiocyanate and indole compounds, which block cancer-causing substances and slow tumor growth. Other cruciferous vegetables, such as cauliflower, cabbage, kale, and collard greens, contain these same compounds.

7.DARK GREEN LEAFY VEGETABLES: like Spinach, chard, kale, collard greens, romaine lettuce, and other dark green leafy vegetables are standout sources of several cancer-fighting substances, including carotenoids. In lab studies, these antioxidant compounds stop cancer cells from growing.

CANCER TREATMENTS

Doctors usually prescribe treatments based on the type of cancer, its stage at diagnosis, and the person's overall health. Below are examples of approaches to cancer treatment:

CHEMOTHERAPY

Chemotherapy: the aims is to kill the cancerous cells with medications that target rapidly dividing cells. The drugs can also help shrink tumors, but the side effects can be severe.

HORMONE THERAPY

Hormone therapy: It involves taking medications that change how certain hormones work or interfere with the body's ability to produce them. When hormones play a significant role, as with prostate and breast cancers, this is a common approach.

IMMUNOTHERAPY

Immunotherapy: uses medications and other treatments to boost the immune system and encourage it to fight cancerous cells. Two examples of these treatments are checkpoint inhibitors and adoptive cell transfer.

PRECISION MEDICINE

Precision medicine or personalized medicine: is a newer, developing approach. It involves using genetic testing to determine the best treatments for a person's particular presentation of cancer. Researchers have yet to show that it can effectively treat all types of cancer, however.

RADIATION THERAPY

Radiation therapy: it uses high-dose radiation to kill cancerous cells. Also, a doctor may recommend using radiation to shrink a tumor before surgery or reduce tumor-related symptoms.

STEM CELL TRANSPLANT

stem cell transplant: can be especially beneficial for people with blood-related cancers, such as leukemia or lymphoma. It involves removing cells, such as red or white blood cells, that chemotherapy or radiation has destroyed. Lab technicians then strengthen the cells and put them back into the body.

SURGERY

Surgery: is often a part of a treatment plan when a person has a cancerous tumor. Also, a surgeon may remove lymph nodes to reduce or prevent the disease's spread.

TARGETED THERAPIES

Targeted therapies: perform functions within cancerous cells to prevent them from multiplying. They can also boost the immune system. Two examples of these therapies are small-molecule drugs and monoclonal antibodies.

Doctors will often employ more than one type of treatment to maximize effectiveness.

HOW TO COPE WITH CANCER DIAGNOSIS

Some tips for coping with a cancer diagnosis include:

- Get the facts about your cancer diagnosis. Keep the lines of communication open with your friends and loved ones, and also, a healthcare provider.
- Anticipate possible physical changes.
- **Consider joining a cancer support group.**
- Find ways to relax, share feelings with loved ones or a counselor, keep a journal, and list pros and cons when making difficult decision.

It takes more time to cope and may involve different strategies depending on the situation, but positive coping strategies can improve emotional well-being and potentially enhance the immune system's response to cancer cell

Many people with cancer have found that practicing relaxation techniques has helped them cope with stress and feel less anxious.

SOME RELAXATION TECHNIQUES THAT MAY BE HELPFUL

The relaxation techniques include:

- SLOW DOWN AND BREATHE: Find a quiet spot where you can be by yourself for a few minutes. Sit down, take a deep breath, and close your eyes. Notice your breath.

- BREATHING AND MUSCLE TENSING: Get into a comfortable position where you can relax your muscles. Close your eyes and clear your mind of distractions. Breathe deeply, at a slow and relaxing pace. Concentrate on breathing deeply and slowly, raising your belly with each breath, rather than just your chest. Next, go through each of your major muscle groups, tensing (squeezing) them for a few seconds and then letting go.

- SLOW RHYTHMIC BREATHING: Stare at an object or shut your eyes and think of a peaceful scene. Take a slow, deep breath. As you breathe in, tense your muscles. As you breathe out, relax your muscles and feel the tension leaving.

- IMAGERY: Create an image in your mind. For example, you may want to think of a place or activity that made you happy in the past.

Explore this place or activity.
Notice how calm you feel.

HOW TO PREVENT CANCER

there are several ways to
reduce the risk of getting
cancer. Some of these include
maintaining a healthy
lifestyle, avoiding exposure to
known cancer-causing
substances, and taking
medicines or vaccines that can
prevent cancer from
developing. Between 30-50%

of all cancer cases are
preventable.

. Some tips to reduce your
risk of cancer include not
using tobacco, eating a
healthy diet, maintaining a
healthy weight and being
physically active, limiting
alcohol consumption, and
getting regular cancer
screenings.

WHAT QUR'AN SAYS ABOUT ENDURING DURING HARDSHIP

Patience is one of the most important actions of the heart mentioned in the Qur'an. Sabr literally means "enduring," "bearing," resisting pain, suffering, and difficulty," and "dealing calmly with problems."

Here are some verses from the Holy Quran on patience:

- "Be patient [steadfast]: God does not let the rewards of

those who do good go to waste" (Quran, 11:115)

Allah says in the Quran: "Verily, We shall put you to test with some fear and hunger, and with some loss of wealth, lives, and offspring. And (o Muhammad) convey good tidings to those who are patients, who say when inflicted by hardship, 'verily we are of God and verily to Him shall we return'. Upon them is the blessings of Allah and His mercy.

And also, the hadith says;

"Abu Sa'id and Abu Hurairah (may Allah be pleased with

them) reported that the Prophet (peace be upon him) said: "Never a believer is stricken with a discomfort, an **illness**, an anxiety, a grief or mental worry or even the pricking of a thorn but Allah will expiate his sins on account of his **patience**". (Al-Bukhari and Muslim)

WHAT BIBLE SAYS ABOUT PATIENCE

The Bible has a lot to say about patience. Patience is

considered a virtue and a fruit of the Spirit. It is characterized by the ability to face trying, hard, or annoying experiences without getting angry, upset, or lashing out. Impatience is considered a form of unbelief and can tempt people to give up or make rash decisions. The opposite of impatience is a deepening, ripening, peaceful willingness either to wait for God where you are in the place of obedience or to persevere at the pace, he allows on the road of obedience.

CONCLUSION

All glory and thanks be to almighty God. We have seen all possible ways to protect ourselves from cancer disease. people are suffering from cancer but I pray with this book you will know about what will harm your health and avoid it.

Please if you see any mistake or **correction** please help me and leave a review for me so that I will not repeat my mistakes again coz this is my first book.

www.ingramcontent.com/pod-product-compliance
Lightning Source LLC
Chambersburg PA
CBHW071939010626
45794CB00025B/2570